IT'S YOUR LIFE – AVOIDING HARMFUL CHEMICALS IN YOUR FOOD

Professor Norman Ratcliffe

A catalogue record for this book is available from the British Library

ISBN: 978-1-907962-57-8

Published by Cranmore Publications

www.cranmorepublications.co.uk

This book is dedicated to my parents whose undying faith in my academic capabilities allowed me to pursue a scientific career. My gratitude also goes to my sister, Teri King, whose success as an author and constant encouragement and advice were such sources of inspiration. Thanks too to my many friends for tolerating so many mealtime discussions on health and diet as well as the unsolicited advice given to them!

Finally, I wish to thank Dr. Duncan McLaren of Swansea Metropolitan University for his outstanding enthusiasm and imagination during creation of sections of this book as well as Doreen Montgomery of Rupert Crew Ltd for her patient and helpful comments of the manuscript.

"IT'S YOUR LIFE"

THE AUTHOR

- **Professor Norman Ratcliffe** is a founder member of a team that recently discovered a new antibiotic potentially capable of curing MRSA and *Clostridium difficile*. This work was presented to Prince Phillip at St. James's Palace, London and was the subject of major media attention in the UK on ITV News and in many leading newspapers, including the Wall Street Journal, around the World. He is a Fellow of the Royal Society of Medicine and has previously run a "Health Alert" blood-testing company. He has published over 200 books and research papers on immunology, cancer invasion, influenza, tropical diseases and MRSA. He played squash for Wales, ran the London Marathon at the age of 50 and works-out regularly in the gym.

- **Professor Ratcliffe** retired recently after 25 years as a University Research Professor. He decided to finally complete "It's Your Life" after 5 years work in order to help the many people who are confused about health and fitness issues and who have constantly been asking his advice.

"IT'S YOUR LIFE"

THE SERIES

Professor Norman Ratcliffe's comprehensive book on health is: *It's Your Life: End the confusion from inconsistent health advice:*

www.cranmorepublications.co.uk/6

This book will often be referred to as IYL. Alongside this comprehensive book there is a series of smaller *It's Your Life: End the confusion from inconsistent health advice* books; this book is the second in the series. The aim of the series is to give advice to people in specific areas; all of the areas covered in the series are also included in IYL. The series is as follows:

It's Your Life – A Healthy Diet Made Easy

www.cranmorepublications.co.uk/61

It's Your Life – Avoiding Harmful Chemicals in Your Food

www.cranmorepublications.co.uk/62

It's Your Life – Avoid the Cocktail Effect of Harmful Chemicals in Your Body

www.cranmorepublications.co.uk/63

It's Your Life – Vitamins and Supplements For All Ages

www.cranmorepublications.co.uk/64

It's Your Life – Exercise For All Ages

www.cranmorepublications.co.uk/65

The main advice arising from IYL has also been summarised in:

117 Health Tips: A quick guide for a healthy life

www.cranmorepublications.co.uk/7

Contents

Chapter 1

IS OUR FOOD SAFE?

Are Pesticide Residues Present In Our Food?

Are Organic Foods Safer?

If you just want to know which foods contain the highest and lowest rates of pesticide residue contamination then go to pages 52 - 62 for a summary of "safe" foods.

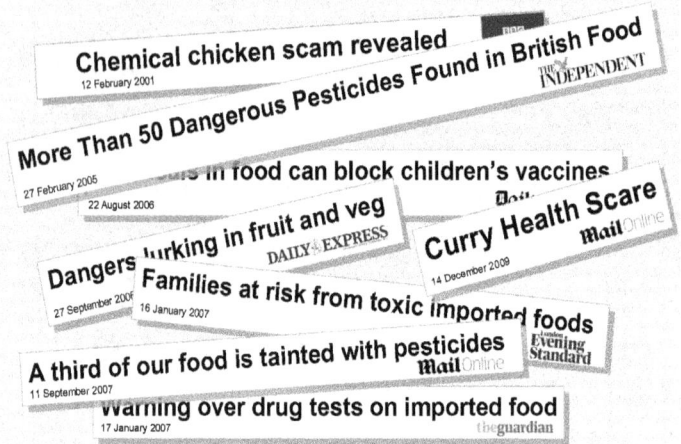

Chemical chicken scam revealed
12 February 2001

More Than 50 Dangerous Pesticides Found in British Food
THE INDEPENDENT
27 February 2005

...s in food can block children's vaccines
22 August 2006

Dangers lurking in fruit and veg
DAILY EXPRESS

Curry Health Scare
Mail Online
14 December 2009

Families at risk from toxic imported foods
27 September 2006   16 January 2007

A third of our food is tainted with pesticides
Mail Online
London Evening Standard
11 September 2007

Warning over drug tests on imported food
17 January 2007
theguardian

As far as our food is concerned, most people are suffering from **"expert opinion overload"**. Almost daily, there are articles in the press and on the radio and television talking about food quality and safety. Recent headlines are shown above.

In addition, a large number of UK organizations, set up for monitoring the safety and quality of our food, seem to be publishing reports almost daily. Thus, we have:

- The Department of Health
- The Food Standards Agency
- The Pesticides Safety Directorate
- The Pesticides Residues Committee
- The Soil Association
- The Food Commission
- The Advisory Committee on Pesticides
- The Committee on Mutagenicity of Chemicals in Food, Consumer Products and the Environment.
- The Pesticide Action Network.
- The British Nutrition Foundation
- The World Wildlife Fund etc, etc.

Unfortunately, as far as food safety is concerned, the opinions of the experts, the stories in the press and the reports from the above organizations are often contradictory. The end result is **CONFUSION** which:

MAY REDUCE PUBLIC TRUST IN FOOD SAFETY IN TERMS OF BOTH CHEMICAL POLLUTION AND HYGIENE

- This chapter is mainly concerned with the safety of our food from chemical residues resulting from the use of chemicals to control pests.

- Subjects such as the nutritional value of food produced by intensive conventional farming and the role of vitamins and supplements are dealt with in Chapters 7 and 8 of IYL.

PUBLIC CONCERN OVER FOOD SAFETY

- A study, during June/July 2006 in the USA by Michigan State University's Food Safety Policy Centre, of over 1,014 people showed that 70% are concerned about pesticide and chemical residues while about 50% are concerned about antibiotics/hormones and additives/preservatives in food (see reference 16b).

- In the UK, public trust in food safety has been eroded following the BSE (early 1990s) and Foot and Mouth (2001) outbreaks, as well as by concern over Genetically Modified (GM) foods (1999), the Sudan I scare in Worcester Sauce (2005) and, more recently, Bird Flu and the mass slaughter of turkeys (2007).

- Previously, over 25% of the UK public believed that food is becoming more risky with particular concern over additives (see reference 17). In a European survey, concerns about pesticide levels in food were rated at the top end of the so-called "worry scale" (see reference 18). Despite reassurances about food safety, a recent UK poll showed that 59% of people interviewed were still worried about contamination of food and drink with pesticides (see reference 19).

- The public, however, does have an increase in trust for the **Food Standards Agency (FSA)** although only 34 % would consult the FSA for information on food safety and 26% for healthy eating **(www.food.gov.uk/).**

- It is obvious that many people are **TOTALLY FED-UP AND CONFUSED** with the constant and inconsistent expert and media advice about food safety and have little idea as to what to believe. The situation is bad enough to have been the butt of jokes on the Terry Wogan Radio 2 show.

- How often do you hear the comment "If you listened to the experts **you wouldn't eat anything"?** Understandably, people may find it difficult to know what to do to avoid the exposure to harmful chemicals in their food.

- Regarding the chemical contamination of food, sometimes, **the appropriate scientific study has not been undertaken** or, if it has, the results have been analysed variably by different organisations. Thus, expert agreement regarding pesticide safety levels may differ significantly.

To ordinary people, the fact that **scientific opinion can disagree widely,** even over the same set of experimental results, is surprising. One good example is the debate between the UK's Pesticide Residues Committee and scientists at the University of Liverpool **over levels of risk from pesticide residues in food** (see reference 20).

In the light of the contradictory and incomplete evidence about the potential harm of chemical pesticides, let us briefly look at some of the important issues of pesticide safety in food and arrive at an unbiased conclusion as to the **safest and most sensible ways of feeding our families.**

WHAT ARE THE FACTS?

Figure 1. Showing the origin of chemical residues in our food

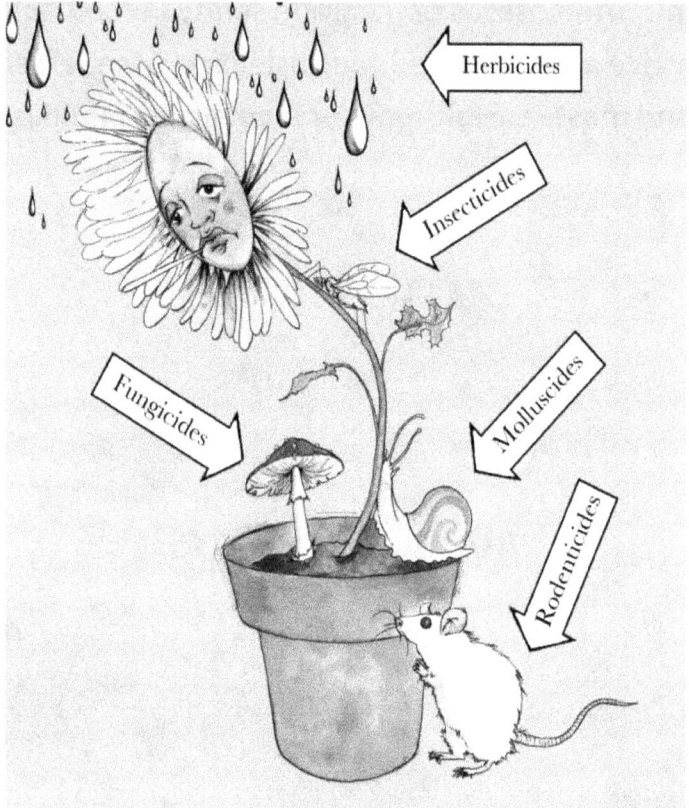

Pesticides are groups of chemicals used to control pests attacking our food crops. The results of the use of these pesticides are not entirely bad and it has been estimated that without the use of artificial nitrogen fertilizers, the World's available fertile land could only support about 60% of the present population (see reference 21). However, with the incidences of some diseases, such as cancers and allergies, increasing at alarming rates, it is time to rectify the environmental damage caused by excessive and poorly controlled use of chemical pesticides. With this aim as a priority, scientists are developing integrated pest management (IPM) programmes, minimising the use of chemicals and reducing the impact on natural animal and plant populations and human health (see references 22, 23).

These pests and the pesticides used (see Figure 1, above) to combat them include:

i. **insects** - insecticide chemicals

ii. **fungal diseases** - fungicides

iii. **weeds** – herbicides

iv.   **slugs and snails** – molluscicides

v.   **rats and mice** – rodenticides

After the crop has been harvested, very small amounts of these chemicals may remain in the food as **chemical residues** that are consumed by both humans and farmed animals. Many of these chemicals are not rapidly eliminated from the body as they dissolve in fatty tissues and then **accumulate in the body** over some considerable time. Examples are DDT, PCBs, dioxins and aldrin that due to their persistence in the environment are often termed **"Persistent Organic Pollutants or POPS"**.

Despite the banning of DDT and other POPS in many countries (Stockholm Convention on POPs, 2001), they are still being found in human tissues. This is due to **bioconcentration** in food chains, through long-term environmental contamination of soils, water and air by pesticide use and by industrial and incineration processes. **As humans are at the top of many foodchains then we may ingest high concentrations of these POPS from fish, meat etc.**

These residual POPs may cause breast and other cancers, suppress the immune system, disturb hormonal functions and pollute human breast milk with unknown short and long-term consequences for babies and infants.

Recently developed and widely used replacement pesticides for POPS include the **organophosphates and carbamates**. These are less environmentally persistent than POPS but are more toxic to humans. Organophosphate insecticides were developed in Germany in the early 1930s but, at the same time, the potential of organophosphates as nerve gases was recognized by the Nazis. They subsequently developed organophosphate nerve gases that are often referred to as:

"Weapons of Mass Destruction"

The effects of exposure to organophosphates and carbamates are similar and include **hormonal disturbances, as well as nervous, behavioural, psychiatric and muscular disorders** such as those experienced by some Gulf War Veterans. Carbamates and organophosphates inhibit the messenger molecule, acetylcholinesterase, between nerve cells, thus preventing nervous transmission and leading to paralysis and even death. Some organophosphates are stored in fatty tissues and cleared slowly from the body. This increases the chances of **enhanced toxicity by the interaction between two or more organophosphates** or with other chemical pollutants. This process is the so-called :

"COCKTAIL EFFECT"

The importance of the cocktail effect is controversial but potentially extremely important and is discussed in detail in Chapter 6 of IYL.

HOW ARE THE LEVELS OF PESTICIDES MONITORED IN OUR FOOD?

Pesticide residues were previously monitored and regulated in our food from 1977 to 2000 by a Government committee. Since 2000, this function has been taken over by an "independent" organization called the **Pesticide Residues Committee (PRC)**. Membership of the PRC, however, is still influenced by Government Ministers and Senior Civil Servants.

The PRC analyses about 4,000 food samples every year for a wide range of pesticides and the results are published four times per year. The types of food monitored are varied from year to year. The detailed reports can be read at **www.pesticides.gov.uk** . The PRC advises the Government as well as the **Food Standards Agency** (FSA, **www.food.gov.uk/**). The FSA is an "independent" Government Department "to protect the public's health and consumer interests in relation to food". The FSA was set up by the Government following the BSE crisis in the UK.

Reports (2005 to 2009) by the PRC on the pesticide residues in food and drink **concluded that the large range of conventionally-produced foods tested were safe** since:

- in about 70% of tested samples no residues were present

- in the remaining 30% of samples with residues, levels of contamination were below statutory safety limits.

Despite these PRC findings, **the public still has deep concerns about food safety** (see above and at **www.foodproductiondaily.com/news**) and the PRC findings have been challenged by many organizations and individuals. One such organization is **Pesticide Action Network, UK** (PAN UK, an "independent, non-profit organization, promoting healthy food, agriculture and an environment") which in 2005 produced its own **"Alternative Pesticide Residues Report"** based on the results of the PRC reports of 2000 to 2005 in which the pesticide residues of common foods were analysed (see reference 24).

There are particular worries about the possible effects of pesticide residues in food on the delicate and rapidly growing bodies of babies and young children. In 1996, the USA National Academy of Science confirmed that any health risks of such chemicals would be magnified in the young (see details in Chapter 6 of IYL, "The Cocktail Effect").

Useful reference for latest reports on food safety is:

www.foodproductiondaily.com/news

The Best and Worst Foods for Pesticide Content are Shown in Tables 1 to 3, below

NB. These Tables are taken from data in the Pesticide Residues Committee (PRC) reports of 2005-2009. In Tables 1 and 2, testing on pears, peaches, nectarines, apples (commonly eaten unpeeled) and also, for some reason, papaya, grapefruits, bananas, oranges, pineapples, lemons, citrus fruits, mangoes, melons, pineapples and probably kiwi, as well as root vegetables was carried out **WITHOUT PEELING or TRIMMING**. Thus, the contamination rates for most of this latter unpeeled produce are not included in Tables 1 and 2 since we do not eat bananas, pineapples etc with their skins on! Furthermore, much evidence shows that peeling/trimming, together with washing and cooking (see references 25-27), removes most of the pesticide contamination. This is confirmed in Tables 1 and 2 since tinned pineapples and mandarins (with peels removed) as well as shelled peas have very low contamination rates in contrast to the unpeeled fruits (90%+ contamination) and peas with pods (60%+). The USA Environmental Protection Agency (EPA) believes that the majority of pesticide residues are in the skins of fruits and vegetables and, in contrast to the UK FSA, very sensibly recommends peeling and washing all produce.

Table 1. FRUITS LISTED WITH HIGHEST AND LOWEST PESTICIDE CONTAMINATION RATES

Fruit Tested[1]	Number of Samples Tested	Percentage of Samples with Pesticides	Results with Organic Samples[2]
Strawberries	92	86-94	6 tested 0+
Apricots	50	84	4 tested 0+
Pears[3] **Unpeeled**	181	78-97	3 tested 1+
Peaches and **Nectarines[3]** **unpeeled**	130	76-93	2 tested 0+
Apples **unpeeled [3]**	346	74-94	15 tested 0+
Grapes[4]	306	70-97	5 tested 0+
Raspberries	36	58	0

Blackberries	36	58	0
Cherries	46	48	0
Pomegranates	37	46	0
Nuts	64	42	3 tested 1+
Plums	72	37	3 tested 0+
Kiwi fruit [3?]	90	26-65	6 tested 0+
Avocados	21	24	3 tested 0+
Orange juice [3]	68	18	4 tested 0+
Mandarins (tinned)	18	17	0
Dried fruit [5]	48	17	4 tested 0+
Lychees	16	12.5	0
Papaya [3]	32	unpeeled	0
Grapefruits [3]	18	unpeeled	0

Bananas [3]	44	unpeeled	4 tested 0+
Oranges[3]	156	unpeeled	3 tested 0+
Pineapples [3]	47	unpeeled	1 tested 0+
Lemons[3]	33	unpeeled	2 tested 0+
Mixed citrus fruits[3,6]	72	unpeeled	0
Melon [3]	96	unpeeled	0
Mangoes	48	unpeeled	0
Apple juice[3]	371	7.5	0
Blueberries	49	6	2 tested 0+
Olives	69	6	1 tested 0+
Peaches (tinned[3])	48	4	1 tested 0+
Pineapples (tinned[3])	18	0	0

More than 50% samples contaminated

20 to 49% samples contaminated

Less than 20% samples contaminated

1. Data for these fruits are taken from the Pesticides Residues Committee (PRC) reports of 2000 to 2009.

2. With organic samples, "0" means no organic samples tested while "0+" means none tested had residues.

3. NB: Many of these fruits were over 75-100% contaminated but they were tested **without peeling,** including pears, peaches, apples, papaya, oranges, grapefruits, lemons, bananas, apples, mangoes, melons, pineapples, and probably kiwi too(?). Evidence on page 28 indicates that most pesticide is removed by peeling. The fact that **whole** pineapples and peaches have high rates of pesticide residues, while tinned pineapples and peaches have much lower levels, indicates that most residues are in the skins of the unpeeled fruits.

4. Grapes are particularly high in multiple pesticide residues as they are often attacked by insect and fungal pests and have to be sprayed frequently.

5. Dried fruits are from grapes and include currants, sultanas and raisins.

6. Includes satsumas, clementines, mandarins and tangerines.

- **Note in Table 1 that most organic fruit samples are free of pesticides**

Table 2. VEGETABLES/SALADS LISTED WITH HIGHEST AND LOWEST PESTICIDE CONTAMINATION RATES

Vegetable/Salad Tested [1]	Number of Samples Tested	Percentage of Samples with Pesticides	Results with Organic Samples[2]
Baby salad [3] (bagged)	72	74	2 tested 1+
Cucumber (unpeeled)	74	69-89	22 tested 2+
Peas fresh[4] (edible pods)	46	61	5 tested 0+
Courgettes (unpeeled)	42	55-77	6 tested 0+
Rice (mixed)	70	50	2 tested 0+
Raddishes	18	50	0
Potato chips[5]	48	48	0
Spinach	101	46-55	5 tested 2+
Potato crisps[5]	132	45	3 tested 0+

Tomatoes (fresh) [4]	142	**43-85[6]**	2 tested 0+
Beans (green + speciality)[7]	143	**38-75[6]**	4 tested 0+
Potatoes [8] (unpeeled)	496	**27-64[6]**	18 tested 1+
Lettuce	253	**26-91[6]**	6 tested 0+
Aubergines	71	**23-39**	0
Okra	47	**17**	0
Peppers	178	**15-61[6]**	0
Turnips	36	**14**	1 tested 1+
Beetroot	7	**14**	11 tested 0+
Celery	107	**13-52[6]**	17 tested 0+
Pulses	84	**13**	4 tested 1+
Parsnips[9]	82	**unpeeled**	15 tested 0+

Carrots	89	unpeeled	7 tested 0+
Sweet potatoes	47	unpeeled	0
Brussel sprouts	18	Not trimmed	0
Yams	46	Unpeeled	0
Onions (bulb)	14	Unpeeled	9 tested 0+
Salad onions	24	Unpeeled	0
Garlic	24	Unpeeled	2 tested 1+
Cabbage	91	Not trimmed	5 tested 0+
Mushrooms	155	9	4 tested 1+
Peas (shelled[4] fresh & frozen)	35	6	1 tested 0+
Leeks	67	5-13	5 tested 0+

Fennel	48	**4**	2 tested 0+
Broccoli	48	**4**	3 tested 0+
Pumpkin	39	**3**	9 tested 0+
Asparagus	95	**1**	0
Cauliflower	33	**0**	3 tested 0+
Tomatoes (tinned) [4]	48	**0**	3 tested 0+
Swede	36	**0**	3 tested 0+
Corn on cob	61	**0**	0
Corn/baby	23	**0**	1 tested 0+
Marrows	59	**0**	0
Baked beans	72	**0**	5 tested 0+
Soup (vegetable)	72	**0**	2 tested 0+
Sunflour and Pumpkin seeds	48	**0**	0

More than 50% samples contaminated

20 to 49% samples contaminated

Less than 20% samples contaminated

1. Data for these vegetables/salads are from the Pesticides Residues Committee (PRC) reports of 2000 to 2009.

2. With organic samples, "0" means no organic samples tested while "0+" means none tested had residues.

3. Baby salad in bags is particularly high in numbers of samples contaminated with pesticides. In addition, more than 17 samples had more than one chemical residue.

4. The fact that peas with pods and tomatoes with skins have higher pesticide rates than shelled peas and tinned tomatoes is additional evidence that the skins of fruit and vegetables protect underlying flesh from contamination.

5. High pesticide residues in potato crisps and chips are of concern and very surprising since peels containing much of the contamination are removed prior to crisp and chip production. This elevated level of pesticides in chips and crisps probably arises during cooking since the oil used is constantly refiltered and reused. Thus, since many pesticides dissolve in fats and oil, any residues in the potatoes will gradually leach out during cooking and concentrate in the oil as it is used time and time again. High levels of pesticides will then be transferred back to the chips via the excess oil sticking to them during cooking.

6. The huge variability in contamination rates from 26 to 91% for lettuce and other foods probably results from samples tested derived from plants grown at different times of the year, or obtained from different suppliers/countries, or may be due to improvements in analytical techniques from one year to the next. Note that some vegetables are classified with "Low" (light grey) or "Medium" (medium grey) contamination rates although the upper range of their contamination rates would place them in the "High" or "Medium" ranges eg. Peppers-15 (low) to 61% (high).

7. Green beans, in particular, have fewer samples with residues than the speciality beans (long beans and soy beans).

8. Potato samples include main crop and new potatoes. During growing, potatoes are sometimes sprayed 19 times per season and 90 pesticides have been registered for use on potatoes of which only about 50% can be detected in the laboratory.

9. Root vegetables and cabbage/Brussel sprouts have not been peeled or trimmed so data for these is not included in Table 2.

- **Note in Table 2 that most organic vegetable samples are free of pesticides**

Table 3. OTHER FOODS LISTED WITH HIGHEST AND
LOWEST PESTICIDE CONTAMINATION RATES[1]

Food Tested [1]	Number of Samples Tested	Percentage of Samples with Pesticides	Results with Organic Samples[2]
FISH [3]			
Salmon (farmed)	63	98	3 tested 2+
Trout (farmed)	45	67	0
Salmon (fresh)	35	60	0
Salmon (tinned)	156	24	0
Mackerel	7	14	0
Fish (deep water)	24	8	0
Trout (fresh)	6	0	0
Fish (take away)	48	0	0

Tuna (tinned)	120	0	0
Shellfish [4]	84	0	0
Prawns	48	0	0
MEAT/MEAT PRODUCTS[5]			
Lamb(New Zealand) [6]	14	29	0
Lamb (mainly UK)	97	14	6 tested 0+
Liver	96	2	0
Beef	192	1	3 tested 0+
Sausages	144	1	0
Bacon	54	0	1 tested 0+
Burgers	72	0	0
Chicken	60	0	2 tested 0+
Duck	36	0	0

Kidneys	59	**0**	0
Liver	71	**0**	0
Meats (tinned)	144	**0**	0
Pate (meat)	72	**0**	1 tested 0+
Turkey	107	**0**	0
DAIRY PRODUCE [7]			
Butter	120	**24**	4 tested 0+
Soya milk	60	**8**	6 tested 0+
Cream	189	**1**	1 tested 0+
Cheese (all sorts)	72	**0**	2 tested 0+
Eggs	132	**0**	12 tested 0+
Fromage frais	13	**0**	0
Low fat spreads	96	**0**	2 tested 0+
Milk (whole fat, semi-skimmed and goats)	298	**0**	65 tested 0+

Yoghurt	107	0	11 tested 0+
CEREALS/ **CEREAL PRODUCTS**			
Rye	34	91	0
Bran	119	88	12 tested 0+
Oats	34	85	0
Flour (wheat)	72	72	6 tested 0+
Bread (all types)	143	72	17 tested 0+
Cereal bars	96	68	2 tested 2+
Rice	168	59.5	3 tested 0+
Breakfast Cereals	144	29	3 tested 0+
Popcorn	29	24	3 tested 0+

Noodles (wheat and rice)	48	**19**	2 tested 0+
Rice cakes	48	**6**	11 tested 0+
Pizza	48	**4**	0
Pasta	144	**1**	12 tested 0+
BABY (INFANT) FOODS			
Infant food (cereal)	202	**8**	71 tested 1+
Infant food (fruit and vegetable)	72	**3**	32 tested 0+
Infant food (meat, fish, cheese)	263	**3**	93 tested 0+
Infant formula	72	**0**	2 tested 0+

DRINKS			
Wine	72	56	0
Beer	48	31^8	0
Tea	96	12.5	4 tested 0+
Coffee	108	0	0
Water (bottled)	50	0	0
MISCELLANEOUS			
Herbs	51	53	0
Peanut butter	24	21	1 tested 0+
Chocolate (white)	48	12.5	5 tested 0+
Honey	72	0	6 tested 0+
Marmalade	48	0	2 tested 0+
Mayonnaise	38	0	0

More   than   50%
samples contaminated

20 to 49% samples
contaminated

Less than 20% samples
contaminated

1. Data for these foods are from the PRC reports of 2000 to 2006. Results from more recent 2008-9 reports are similar to those in Table 3.

2. With organic samples "0+" means no samples with residues while "0+" means none tested had residues.

3. Some fish, including tuna, marlin, swordfish and shark, accumulate relatively high levels of heavy metals and pregnant women should avoid these (see, " Mercury levels in fish", page 58).

4. Shellfish includes mussels, oysters, whelks and scallops but not crabs, lobsters and prawns.

5. The results for meat/meat products are for contaminating pesticides but not for artificial hormones and antibiotics, which are both banned in the EU, but often given to animals outside the EU to stimulate growth (see page 59).

6. The origin of pesticides in New Zealand lamb is as a result of persistent organochlorine (eg. DDT) contamination of the environment from past use.

7. Dairy produce should be safe from pesticides, artificial hormones contamination and antibiotics in the UK.

8. With beer DO NOT PANIC!! Pesticides in beer come from the hops but levels are very low (see reference 28).

- **Note, with only two exceptions, that all organic samples are free of pesticides**

OVERALL SUMMARY FROM TABLES 1-3 OF FOODS WITH HIGHEST AND LOWEST PESTICIDE CONTAMINATION RATES

IMPORTANT

COPY THIS LIST AND ATTACH TO NOTICEBOARD OR FRIDGE AS A REMINDER

FRUITS

Lowest rates

↓

- All fruits with peel or skins, such as citrus fruits, bananas, mangoes, pineapples, melons, apples etc, probably have the lowest rates of pesticide contamination **AFTER THE PEEL/SKIN IS REMOVED**.

Highest rates

↓

- In contrast, many "soft" fruits, such as grapes, strawberries, apricots, raspberries, cherries, plums, and peaches as well as unpeeled apples and pears, have the highest rates of pesticide contamination. Most of these are not peeled before eating and pesticides probably bind to the skins.

- Organic fruit is expensive so give priority to organic soft fruit or apples and pears if you eat the skin. Unfortunately, organic soft fruit is expensive so wash non-organic soft fruit (uncut to avoid loss of vitamins) for 30sec to 5 min.

VEGETABLES/SALADS

Lowest rates

↓

- All vegetables that are peeled/podded before eating, such as peas, peeled potatoes, tinned/peeled tomatoes, mushrooms, turnips, parsnips, onions, leeks, carrots, swedes, corn, broad beans, baked beans, etc, probably have the lowest rates of pesticide contamination.

> **These have low
> rates too!**

↓

- Some items with no peel also have low contamination rates, including cabbage, okra, fennel, broccoli, asparagus, cauliflower, and marrows.

Highest rates

↓

- In contrast, items with no peel or unpeeled before use, such as bagged salad, fresh lettuce, celery, aubergines, peas with edible pods, green beans, salad onions as well as unpeeled potatoes, fresh tomatoes, cucumber, peppers and courgettes, have the highest rates of pesticide contamination.

- Organic vegetables are more expensive and often unavailable so always wash and/or trim all non-organic and unpeeled vegetables and salads. **Always buy organic potatoes which are relatively cheap and available.**

- Beware bought chips and crisps since these may have high pesticide rates from contaminated cooking oil. Make your own chips if you must.

OTHER FOODS

Lowest rates

↓

- Generally, fish and shellfish (except fresh and farmed salmon, and farmed trout), all meats (except New Zealand Lamb), dairy products, pizzas, pastas, baby foods, tea, coffee, bottled water, chocolate, honey, marmalade, and mayonnaise, have the lowest rates of pesticide contamination.

Highest rates

↓

- In contrast, cereals and cereal products, such as wheat flour, rye, bran, oats, rice, bread, cereal bars, and breakfast cereals, have high rates of pesticide contamination.

- Organic foods are more expensive so **IT IS MOST IMPORTANT TO BUY ORGANIC BREAD, PORRIDGE, FLOUR AND CEREAL BARS.**

Mercury levels in fish

↓

- Many fish also contain traces of mercury so that children under 16 as well as pregnant women and women planning pregnancy should avoid shark, marlin and swordfish and limit themselves to two fresh tuna steaks per week. Tinned tuna is safer. Mercury may affect the nervous system of the unborn baby and young children. Cod, haddock and plaice are fine.

Antibiotics in meat

↓

- Although meats and dairy produce have low rates of pesticide contamination, antibiotics are sometimes added to animal feeds outside the EU and these may contaminate imported foods. It is better to buy UK produce if you are certain of the origin. Organic meat and dairy produce is readily available but expensive. Marks and Spencer and Sainsbury's specialise in quality meats and poultry and sometimes are as cheap as other higher volume supermarkets.

OVERALL SUMMARY AND WHICH ORGANIC FOODS ARE MOST IMPORTANT TO BUY

1. Generally, fruits and vegetables once skinned, peeled, shelled or trimmed will probably have low pesticide contamination levels so organic is unnecessary.

2. Most soft fruits (but not blueberries) have high pesticide levels so wash thoroughly (uncut). Organic grapes and strawberries are available but expensive.

3. Always buy organic apples/pears or peel before eating.

4. Many vegetables, including lettuce, celery, and tomatoes as well as aubergines, peas with edible pods, green beans, and salad onions have high pesticide rates but buying organic is difficult. Again, washing thoroughly will help. Locally grown produce will also have lower pesticide levels.

5. Always buy organic potatoes, if you eat the skins, as these are available and cheap.

6. Many other foods like meats and dairy produce have low pesticide levels so organic are unnecessary but trim off excess fat.

7. It is most important to buy organic and wholemeal bread, cereals, cereal bars, porridge and flour.

NOTE: Many of the above organic items are not regularly available or are too expensive at UK supermarkets in which case concentrate on buying **organic potatoes, bread, cereals (and cereal products) and porridge** most of which are usually present on the shelves.

CHAPTER 2

IS OUR FOOD SAFE?

ADDITIVES

Preservatives, Colourants and Sweeteners

If you just want to know the dangerous ones and how to avoid them go to Section 3 (below)

- **Practically all the food we buy contains additives**

- **Do not panic as advice is given below on "how to avoid the most dangerous additives"**

- **It makes sense to reduce the number of chemicals eaten**

IN OUR FOOD

- There are over 300 different food additives approved for use by the European Union (all with E numbers)

- Around 2600 flavourings are in use in Europe

- Numerous vitamins and minerals are added

- Artificial trans fats are used

Figure 1. Representing the factory processing of our food and the robotic addition of additives on the conveyor belt

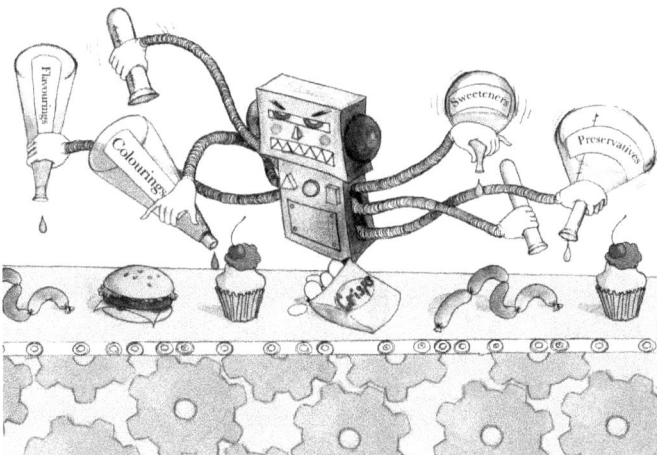

SECTION 1: EXAMPLES OF ADDITIVES PRESENT IN COMMON FOODS AND DRINKS

1. **Muller Light Strawberry, fat-free yoghurt, 200g**
   strawberries (10%)

   beetroot red (E162) and carmine (E120), (colours)

   flavourings (not identified)

   aspartame (E951), (sweetener)

   citric acid (E330) and sodium citrate (E331), (acidity regulators)

   gelatine (E441), (gelling agent)

   Total additives = at least 8

2. SPAR Whole Orange Squash
orange from concentrate (10%!)

potassium sorbate (E202) and sodium metabisulphate (E223), (preservatives)

beta-carotene (E160a), (colour)

malic acid (E296) + others (flavourings)

aspartame (E951) and sodium saccharin (E 954), (sweeteners)

carboxymethylcellulose (E466), (stabilizer)

citric acid (E330) and sodium citrate (E331), (acidity regulators)

Total additives = at least 9

3. Diet Coke
   carbonated water

   caramel (E150a), (colour)

   citric acid (E330), (flavouring and preservative)

   caffeine + others? (flavourings)

   phosphoric acid (E338), (flavouring and acidity regulator)

   aspartame (E951) and acesulfame k (E950), (sweeteners)

Total additives = just water mixed with 5-6 chemicals

WHAT DO YOU THINK OF THE FOLLOWING STATEMENT?

"Soft drinks are an enjoyable source of fluid, which is essential to good health. In combination with a varied diet and regular activity, soft drinks can provide a refreshing and positive contribution to everyday living" from Coca Cola (www.cokeeducation.co.uk).

Comment: Surely, a chemical mixture is not to be preferred to plain water or a 100% pure fruit drink with no additives?

4. **Hot Dog 2 Pack (Snack Express)**

   a. roll

   calcium propionate (E282). (preservative)

   esters of fatty acids (E471, E 472e), (emulsifiers)

   vitamin C (E300), (flour treating agent)

b. sausage

sodium nitrite (E250), (preservative)

vitamin C (E300), (antioxidant)

citric acid (flavouring and preservative)

monosodium glutamate (E621), (flavour enhancer)

potassium polymetaphosphate (E452), (stabiliser)

glucono-delta-lactone (E575), (acidity regulator)

c. ketchup

potassium sorbate (E202), (preservative)

flavouring (not identified)

d. mustard

flavouring (not identified)

Total additives = 13 including:

3 preservatives, 1 antioxidant, 4 flavourings, 2 emulsifiers, 1 stabiliser, 1 acidity regulator, 1 flour treating agency plus 3.6 g salt (over half of recommended daily allowance = RDA level).

Remember, many similar and even worse examples can easily be found on any supermarket shelf. For example, a small Nutrigrain Soft Bake Bar has over 16 such additives. **Unfortunately, additives are often associated with the sweets, biscuits, cakes and soft drinks eaten and drunk by our children.**

SECTION 2: TYPES OF ADDITIVES AND THEIR ROLES IN OUR FOOD

Additives approved of by the European Union are labelled on food either by name or have been given an "E" number. In Europe, the "E" numbers indicate that the additives have apparently been tested for safety by the EU (see reference 29 for a full list).

The E numbers of a large number of additives generally fall into the following groups:

- Food colourants are usually E100 to E180.

- Preservatives are mainly E200 to E285.

- Antioxidants are mainly E300 to E321.

- Many thickeners, emulsifiers, stabilisers and gelling agents are included in E400 to E495.

- Many artificial sweeteners are included in E420, E421 and E950-E968.

- There are many other additives with E numbers, such as anti-caking agents and acidity regulators, with numbers going as high as E1500. The numbering scheme misses out many numbers including the 700-800s etc.

1. COLOURANTS (42 approved)

These maintain the natural colour lost in food during processing or storage and also increase the attractiveness of food to the consumer. They are also used to colour artificial "foods" such as sweets or candy and include both natural and synthetic chemical dyes. **Artificially coloured foods are often targeted at children and some sweets, biscuits and desserts may contain multiple colourants**. There is concern that children consume much higher doses of colourants than adults and one study has estimated that they may take in 35-40 different doses of over 12 different colours per day! There are worries (see Section 3 "Safety Concerns", below) about the effects upon children's behaviour of some of the **synthetic azo dyes** commonly used in sweets, soft drinks and ice cream and particularly:

i. Tartrazine (E102)

ii. Quinoline yellow (E104)

iii. Sunset yellow (E110)

iv. Carmoisine or **Azorubine** (E122)

v. Ponceau 4R or **Cochineal Red A** (E124)

vi. Allura Red (E129)

2. PRESERVATIVES (37 approved)

These prevent spoiling of food during transportation and storage. Older preservation techniques include boiling, refrigeration and pickling, as well as the use of salt and sugar. More recently, chemical preservatives have been introduced and are designed to kill bacteria and moulds contaminating food. There are, however, Safety Concerns (see, Section 3, below) in the use of some of these chemicals. These chemicals are designed to increase the shelf-life of food and include:

i. Sulphur dioxide (E220) for dried fruit

ii. Nitrites (E249, 250) and **Nitrates** (E251, 252) with bacon, sausages, ham, corned beef and nearly all cooked meats

iii. Benzoates (E210-213) and **Sorbates** (E200, E201, 202 and 203) are very widely used, especially in soft drinks such as carbonated, squash and still drinks as well as wine making

3. ANTIOXIDANTS (17 approved)

These include natural antioxidants as well as synthetic antioxidants and are added to food as preservatives to inhibit microbial activity. They also prevent food spoilage caused by exposure to oxygen as seen with the browning of cut potatoes and apples. Two naturally-occurring antioxidants often used are:

i. Vitamin C (ascorbic acid, E300)

ii. Vitamin E (tocopherols, E306)

These vitamin antioxidants are also widely used in foods containing fats or oils to prevent discoloration and odours resulting from contact with oxygen or enzymes which turn fats such as butter rancid (=oxidation). Oxidation of the fats and oils is inhibited by Vitamins C and E that interact with (scavenge) the oxygen. More controversial (see, Section 3 "Safety Concerns", below) is the use of petroleum-based and synthetic antioxidants such as:

iii. Butylated hydroxyanisole (BHA, E320)

iv. Butylated hydroxytoluene (BHT, E321)

4. THICKENERS, EMULSIFIERS, STABILIZERS, ANTI-CAKING AGENTS, ACIDITY REGULATORS, GELLING AGENTS etc (205 approved)

These, for example, thicken soups, maintain mayonnaise in suspension, and prevent lumps forming in salt and flour. Examples are:

i. Pectin (E449) **and Gelatin** (E441) for thickening and stabilizing foods, such as desserts and ice cream allowing them to set and the components to remain in suspension

ii. Lecithin (E322) is an emulsifier and maintains oil, vinegar and water mixed together in suspension in mayonnaise and salad dressings

iii. Calcium silicate (E552) **and silicon dioxide** (E551) are anti-caking agents used to maintain the free flow and prevent lumps forming in powdered food like salt and drinking chocolate

5. ARTIFICIAL SWEETENERS (15 approved)

These are used widely to replace sugar as they contain fewer calories. They are present in so-called "low calorie", "lite" and "low sugar" biscuits, sweets, chewing gum, jams, fizzy and soft drinks, and diet desserts such as yoghurts. The following commonly used, so-called "intense sweeteners" are even sweeter than sugar itself and used at very low concentrations:

i. Acesulfame-K (E950)

ii. Aspartame (E951)

iii. Cyclamate or Cyclamic Acid (E952)

iv. Saccharin (E954)

v. Sucralose (E955)

There has been widespread debate over the safety of these intense sweeteners, especially for children, as they are widely used as sugar substitutes in drinks such as "Coca-Cola Zero", "Fanta", "Sprite", "Dr Pepper" and "Lilt" as well as other soft drinks and squashes (see, Section 3, "Safety Concerns", below).

Other artificial sweeteners include:

vi. Sorbitol (E420)

vii. Mannitol (E421)

These are about 60% as sweet as sugar, and used in similar amounts to sugar, but contain fewer calories and are particularly useful for dieters and for sweetening foods for diabetics.

6. FLAVOUR ENHANCERS AND FLAVOURINGS

i. Flavour enhancers are added to food and drinks to bring out their natural taste. Simple examples used commonly are salt and vinegar. Another example is **monosodium glutamate** (MSG, E621) which is widely used in Chinese food, barbecue sauces, snack foods, frozen dinners and stock cubes.

ii. Flavourings are added to a wide range of foods to give a particular taste or smell. Flavourings can be natural or artificial and at present there are 2600 flavourings in use in the European Union. These additives have not been given E numbers. The European Food Safety Authority (**www.efsa.europa.eu**) intends to evaluate the safety of all flavourings and produce a list authorized for use in the EU. Unfortunately, **food labels often indicate the use of flavourings but fail to name them** so that tighter controls are required (see, Section 3, "Safety Concerns" below, for both MSG and flavourings).

7. NUTRITIONAL ADDITIVES

These include vitamins A, B, C and D, as well as iron, calcium and zinc which are added to fortify some bread, cereals, flour, milk and margarine. Many foods are fortified in the UK and readers should check the labels, particularly of children's sugary cereals and drinks, and realize that these foods are often fortified because of their poor nutritional value.

TRANS FATS (HYDROGENATED FATS)

These are artificially made by passing hydrogen through liquid vegetable oils until they solidify. By this method, margarines were developed as alternative spreads to butter. The food industry readily adopted them as they are cheap padding agents for more expensive foods and also improve both the texture and shelf-life of food.

- However, **trans fats in many studies have been shown to be linked to the development of coronary heart disease** (see reference 30)

- Trans fats are found in fast (junk) food such as chicken nuggets, french fries, as well as in fritters, potato crisps, pizza, ice-cream, puddings, pies, cakes and cake mixes, biscuits, doughnuts, gravy and sauce mixes, confectionery and many other processed foods, including some children's high-sugar breakfast cereals. They are also present in restaurant food and can be formed too by repeatedly re-heating cooking oil.

SECTION 3: SAFETY CONCERNS

The European Food Safety Authority (EFSA) is responsible for the safety evaluation of additives for the EU while in the UK the Food Standards Agency (FSA) monitors the safety and use of food additives. The Food and Drug Administration (FDA) controls the use of food additives in the USA.

Despite the fact that food additives in Europe have been given "E" numbers, indicating that they have apparently been tested for safety and approved by the EU, **frequent concerns have arisen as to the wisdom of adding so many chemicals to our food.**

Many people are concerned about food additives and are probably not reassured by Government Agencies. Who can ever forget the BSE crisis and the graphic assurances by the minister in charge that our beef was safe?

On the other hand, it is necessary to maintain a balanced view since many food additives are naturally-occurring substances and harmless, such as the colourants, paprika (E160c), lycopene (E160d) and curcumin (E100). Some food additives, such as salt (within the 6gm limit per day) and vinegar (contains acetic acid, E260), have even been used for hundreds of years with no adverse effects reported.

There is no doubt that additional careful testing of food additives is required as indicated by recent findings that a cocktail of artificial colourants together with the preservative, sodium benzoate, increases hyperactivity in children (McCann and colleagues, The Lancet, Vol. 370, pages 1560 - 1567, 2007, reference 31). Previously, in the 1980s, it had been reported that there was no evidence that such colourants or food additives caused hyperactivity in children.

MAIN FOOD ADDITIVES OF CONCERN

1. COLOURANTS E100-180 may trigger hives, urticaria, asthma and generalized allergic reactions. Of particular concern are the so-called **"azo dyes"** which are widely used in hundreds of food products and medicines. Azo dyes are **synthetic colourants** extracted from crude oil but in the body some:

- **May be cancer-forming**

- **Are also suspected of triggering allergies and behaviour/learning problems in children such as attention deficit hyperactivity disorder (ADHD)**

- **As well as allergies such as asthma, itching, rhinitis and stomach upsets occur especially in those with aspirin sensitivity/allergy.**

Following the McCann and colleagues study published in The Lancet, 2007 (see, above = reference 31), the Foods Standard Agency called for a voluntary ban by the end of 2009 on the first 6 dyes in the list in Table 1 (below). The EU also requires food containing these dyes to be labelled "may have an adverse effect on activity and attention of children".

Major shops in the UK, including Tesco, Marks and Spencer, Iceland, Co-op and Asda, either do not use these six colourants or have removed them from their OWN BRAND products.

Food manufacturers also producing foods free of these six colourants include Unilever, Nestle, Cadbury, Trebor Bassett, Heinz (Heinz, Weight Watchers, HP, and Lea & Perrins), Worldfoods, Vimto Soft Drinks (Sunkist, Panda and Vimto) as well as McDonald's OWN BRAND food and drinks.

THERE ARE 16 COLORANTS OF CONCERN [*]:

i. **Tartrazine** (E102)

ii. **Quinoline Yellow** (E104)

iii. **Sunset Yellow** also called **Orange Yellow S** (E110)

iv. **Carmoisine** also called **Azorubine** (E122)

v. **Ponceau 4R** also called **Cochineal Red A** (E124)

vi. **Allura Red** (E129)

vii. **Amaranth** (E123)

viii. **Erythrosine** (E127)

ix. **Red 2G** (E128)

x. **Patent Blue V** (E131)

xi. **Indigo Carmine** (E132)

xii. **Brilliant Blue FCF** (E133)

xiii. **Ammonia Caramel** (150c)

xiv. **Brilliant Black BN** also called **Black PN** (E151)

xv. **Brown FK** (E154)

xvi. **Brown HT or Chocolate Brown HT** (E155)

 * For a list of permitted food colourants in the
EU see reference 32

**Figure 2. Showing a bowl of sweets and the E numbers of
colourants used as additives**

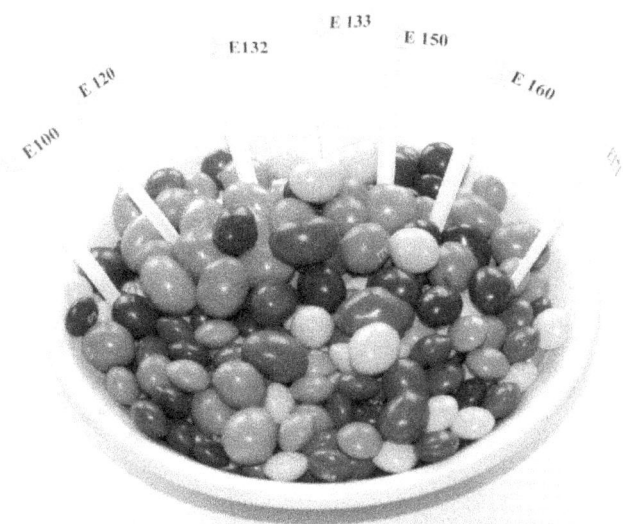

Avoiding Harmful Chemicals in Your Food

Table 1.   COLOURANT ADDITIVES CAUSING SAFETY CONCERNS

Colourant Name	Present in which foods	Safety Concerns and Possible Health Effects
The first 6 colourants are the azo dyes included in the McCann and colleagues (2007) research[1] and linked to hyperactivity in children. Remove these from the diet.		
i. Tartrazine (E102)	Yellow, in soft drinks, sweets, ices, jams, cereals, cake mixes, mustard, yoghurts, some package soups, and tinned foods	Linked to hyperactivity and ADHD[2] in children, as well as allergies associated with itching, rhinitis, migraine, asthma etc. Banned in Austria, Germany and Norway

ii. Quinoline Yellow (E104)	Soft drinks, cough sweets, ices, scotch eggs, chewing gum, and smoked haddock. Also, in lipstick and children's medicines	Linked to hyperactivity and ADHD[2] in children, as well as allergies, such as dermatitis. May damage genes and cause cancer. Banned in Australia, Japan, Norway and USA
iii. Sunset Yellow (E110)	Soft drinks, sweets, ices, jellies, trifle, apricot jam, marzipan, lemon curd, Swiss roll, hot chocolate and packet soups. Also, breadcrumbs, cheese sauce, canned fish, and children's medicines	Linked to hyperactivity and ADHD[2] in children and allergic reactions and can result in stomach upsets, nettle rash etc. Sometimes contaminated with Sudan I, a banned cancer forming azo dye. Banned in Canada, Japan, Scandinavia and USA

iv. Carmoisine (Azorubine) (E122)	Red dye in soft drinks, sweets, jellies, marzipan, yoghurt, cheese-cakes and children's medicines	Linked to hyperactivity and ADHD[2] in children and allergic reactions such as skin rash in asthmatics. Banned in Japan, Norway, Sweden and USA
v. Ponceau 4R (E124)= Cochineal Red A	Red dye in some drinks, sweets, cakes, dessert toppings, salami, salad dressings, cheesecakes and trifles	Linked to hyperactivity and ADHD[2] in children and can produce bad reactions in asthmatics. Regarded as cancer-forming in animals. Banned in Finland Norway and USA
vi. Allura Red (E129)	In soft drinks, sweets, biscuits, cereals, condiments and medicines	Linked to hyperactivity and ADHD[2] in children, and may produce bad reactions in people allergic to aspirin. Linked with cancer in mice. Banned in Austria, Belgium, France, Germany, Scandinavia and Switzerland

The following colourants include azo dyes, but were not tested in the McCann and colleagues research[1]. They may also cause behavioural/learning problems in children, as well as allergic reactions and even cancer in adults but proof is sometimes incomplete. All food colourants must now be labelled. Colorants E100 - E180 may trigger hives, urticaria, asthma and generalized allergic reactions.

vii. Amaranth (E123)	Purple-red azo dye in some blackcurrant and red soft and alcoholic drinks, ice creams, jams, jellies, tinned fruit, trifle, cake mixes, prawns, gravy granules, soups and medicines	Linked to allergies, asthma, eczema and hyperactivity in children. Numerous studies link it to cancer in laboratory animals, birth defects, stillbirths, sterility and early foetal death. Banned in Austria, Norway, Russia, United States, and with restricted use in France and Italy (caviar only).

viii. Erythrosine **(E127)**	Pink-red, non-azo, synthetic, coal tar dye in sweets, biscuits, cakes, glace cherries, strawberries and rhubarb, packet desserts, spreads and patés, processed cooked meat	Potentially causing thyroid problems and reduces sperm count in animals, potential factor in breast cancer. Recommended for banning in USA
ix. Red 2G **(E128)**	Azo dye found in some breakfast sausages and burgers	Potentially cancer-forming. The EFSA[3] banned it's use in 2007 including in UK. Already banned in many countries such as Norway and USA
x. Patent Blue **V** **(E 131)**	A non-azo, synthetic, coal tar dye not widely used in foods but in sweets, occasional soft drink and scotch	Linked to allergies, nettle rash, itching, low blood pressure and occasional serious allergic shock. Banned in Australia, Japan, USA,

	eggs. Also, in plaque disclosing tablets and injected to trace blood vessels	Norway, New Zealand
xi. Indigo Carmine (E132)	Blue, non-azo, synthetic dye, derived from coal tar. Found in sweets, ice cream, baked goods, confectionary, biscuits, as well as tablets and capsules	In people such as asthmatics, may cause nausea, vomiting, high blood pressure, skin rashes, breathing problems and other allergic reactions. Banned in Norway.
xii. Brilliant Blue FCF (E133)	Non-azo, synthetic dye from coal tar. Often found in sweets, ice cream, dairy products, drinks, tinned peas, cosmetics and soaps	Hyperactive Children's Support Group (HACSG)[4] recommends elimination from children's diets. Cancer induction unproven? EU approved. Banned previously in Austria , Belgium, France, Germany Norway, Sweden and Switzerland

xiii. Ammonia Caramel (E150c)	Non-azo dye widely used in chocolates, ice cream, soft drinks, beer, wine, whiskey bakery goods, pickles, sauces, snacks	Possible allergen. Reports of adverse effects on hyperactivity, and toxicity to stomach, liver, reproduction and blood need confirmation
xiv. Brilliant Black BN (E151)	Azo dye found in soft drinks, flavored milk, sweets, ice cream, blackcurrant cake mixes, food decorations, desserts, jellies, red fruit jams, mustard, brown sauces, fish paste etc	HACSG[4] recommends elimination from children's diets. May damage genes and cause cancer. Banned in Australia, much of Western Europe and USA
xv. Brown FK (E154)	Azo dye found in smoked fish, cooked meat and crisps	Similar concerns to Brilliant Blue (E133), including hyperactivity and ADHD

xvi. Brown HT (E155)	An azo dye found mainly in chocolate flavour cakes.	Similar concerns to Brilliant Blue (E133), including hyperactivity and ADHD[2].

1. McCann and colleagues, The Lancet, Vol. 370, pages 1560 - 1567, 2007, reference 31.

2. ADHD =attention deficit hyperactivity disorder

3. EFSA is the European Food Safety Authority **(www.efsa.europa.eu)**

4. HACSG is the Hyperactive Children's Support Group **(www.hacsg.org.uk)**

BOTTOM LINE ON FOOD COLOURANTS

BE PARTICULARLY CONCERNED FOR
POSSIBLE EFFECTS ON:

- Children - may induce allergies and behavioural effects

- Adults - may induce or aggravate allergies

Note also:

- That many cosmetics and some children's medicines contain azo dyes (see reference 33)

- Manufacturers are removing these colourants from many sweets and medicines although the latter still contain sulphite preservatives (see, Table 2, below)

2/3. PRESERVATIVES AND ANTIOXIDANTS

TABLE 2.   PRESERVATIVE AND ANTIOXIDANT ADDITIVES CAUSING SAFETY CONCERNS

Preservative Name	Present in which Foods	Safety Concerns and Possible Health Effects
i. **Sorbates** **E200-203** Sorbic acid (E200) Sodium sorbate (E201)	Widely used anti-microbial agents, found in soft drinks, sweets, wine, cakes, pies, pickles, salad dressings, sauces, dairy products (not milk drinks), dry	**Generally recognized as safe by** JECFA[1], FDA[2] and the FSA[3]. However, sorbic acid has been shown to interact with nitrite preservative to form low levels of cancer–forming agents but none of these have been shown to

Potassium sorbate (E202) Calcium sorbate (E203)	fruits, fish, beauty /health products etc	transform cells [4]. Sorbic acid may cause skin irritation.
ii. Benzoates **E210-214** Benzoic acid (E210) Sodium benzoate (E211) Potassium benzoate (E212) Calcium benzoate (E213) Ethyl 4-hydroxybenzoate (E214)	Widely used anti-microbial agents, found in soft drinks, sweets, jellies, jams, cakes, pickles, salad dressings, sauces, crisps, child medicines, beauty and health products etc	**Whether sodium benzoate (E211) is safe is controversial.** E211 was mixed with azo dyes in the McCann et al., (2007) study [5] on azo dyes linked to hyperactivity in children. The FSA[3] banned these dyes but not E211. Benzoates may aggravate asthma and allergies and HACSG [6] suggests avoidance. E211 can interact with vitamin C in soft drinks to form the cancer-forming compound, benzene. There is evidence for damage to DNA in cells [7]. Parents should

		prevent children from drinking too many soft drinks with E211 and azo dyes.
iii. Sulphites **E220-228** Sulphur dioxide (E220) Sodium sulphite (E221) Sodium bisulphite (E222) Sodium metabisulphite (E223) Potassium metabisulphite (E224) Calcium sulphite (E226)	Anti-microbial agents, used in soft drinks and fruit juices, jams, sausages, beer, wine, yoghurt, potato products, frozen shellfish, pickles, balsamic vinegar and **often in dried fruits**. In beer and wine but may not be labelled. Also in medicines (including children's), cosmetics, beauty and hair care products.	**Much concern over safety of sulphites. In USA FDA[2] prohibits use on fresh fruit and vegetables** including peeled potatoes to stop browning. Can provoke sneezing, breathing problems etc in asthmatics and even severe shock. Sulphites have been included among the top 10 substances causing allergies. Some antihistamines medicines may contain sodium bisulphite! Some sulphites also destroy vitamin B1 (thiamin). In UK sulphite levels in food above 10mg

Calcium bisulphite (E227) Potassium bisulphate (E228)		per kg or litre should be labelled.
iv. **Nitrites and Nitrates (E249-252)** Potassium nitrite (E249) Sodium nitrite (E250) Sodium nitrate (E 251) Potassium nitrate (E 252)	Antibacterial agents, colour and flavour stabilizers used in cured and smoked meats such as ham, bacon, tongue, hot dogs, corned beef, sausages, salami, luncheon meat, as well as fish. Beware burnt or charred red meat such as crispy fried bacon. Also, present in cosmetics.	**Much media concern for safety of nitrites and nitrates used in cured meats as they can be converted in the body into cancer-forming nitrosamines.** However, it has been estimated that only about 5% of your daily intake of nitrosamines comes from cured meat with most derived from vegetables and drinking water (from nitrates used as fertilizers), cigarette smoke, cars etc. Even so, the EFSA[8] and FSA[3] have reduced the levels of

		potassium and sodium nitrates allowed in meat products. Sodium nitrite may induce hyperactivity and HACSG [6] suggests avoidance. Vitamin C and E may block cancer-forming nitrosamines [9].
v. Butylated hydroxyanisole (BHA) (E 320)	Antioxidant preservative, in UK mainly used in butter, margarine, lard and vegetable oils to prevent them becoming rancid or bad. Also in sweets, cereals, chewing gum, potato chips, meats, nuts, lipstick and eye shadow	**Suspected as a cancer-inducing agent although evidence inconclusive.** May interact in stomach with nitrites to produce cancer-forming compounds. Also, limited evidence of association with allergic or intolerance responses such as asthma and rhinitis. Now being replaced by natural antioxidants such as

		vitamins E and C. Should not be present in infants' food. Banned in Japan and by McDonalds in USA.
vi. **Butylated hydroxytoluene** **(BHT) (E 321)**	See E320, above	See E320, above

1. JECFA is World Health Organisation (WHO) Expert Committee on Food Additives

2. FDA is US Food and Drug Administration **(www.cfsan.fda.gov/~dms/fdsweet.html)**

3. FSA is Food Standards Agency, UK **(www.food.gov.uk)**

4. See reference 34.

5. See reference 31.

6. HACSG is the Hyperactive Children's Support Group (**www.hacsg.org.uk**)

7. See reference 35.

8. EFSA is the European Food Safety Authority (**www.efsa.europa.eu**)

9. See reference 36.

BOTTOM LINE ON CHEMICAL FOOD PRESERVATIVES AND ANTIOXIDANTS

- Sorbates are recognised as the safest group of preservatives.

- Children are particularly vulnerable to the effects of preservatives due to excessive intakes in soft drinks and sweets.

- More "natural" preservatives are now being researched and introduced slowly.

- Levels of some chemical preservatives in food are being reduced by FSA and EFSA legislation.

- Cured meats labelled "naturally cured" or "no added nitrite" may contain nitrite from plant material high in nitrates and used for curing.

- NB: Many cosmetics, beauty and hair products may also contain chemical preservatives.

4. ARTIFICIAL SWEETENERS

The most widely used and those causing safety concerns are included in Table 3, below.

Table 3.   ARTIFICIAL SWEETENERS CAUSING SAFETY
CONCERNS

Sweetener Name	Present in which Foods	Safety Concerns and Possible Health Effects
i. Acesulphame K (E950)	Marketed as "Sunette", "Ace K" and "Sweet One". Used widely in soft drinks such as Diet Coke and alcoholic drinks. Also in sweets, ice cream, desserts, jams, dairy products, baked goods, chewing gum, dressings, body builders' protein drinks, toothpaste,	Acesulphame has been widely tested **and is generally recognized as safe by JECFA[1], FDA[2] and the FSA[3]**. It is approved for use in many countries. There have, however, been adverse reports suggesting cancer-forming properties[4] and suggestions of the need for additional testing[5]. Furthermore, acesulphame, like all artificial sweeteners,

	mouthwash, cosmetics, medicines	may affect the blood sugar and increase food cravings? Banned from young children's products
ii. **Aspartame** **(E951)**	Marketed as "Equal", "Canderel", and "NutraSweet". Found in about 6000 foods Worldwide such as soft drinks, sweets, desserts, chewing gum, dairy products, cakes, biscuits, jams, vitamin and mineral pills, weight-control products, as a substitute for sugar in hot drinks, and in medicines	**Aspartame has been recognized as safe by FDA[2], FSA[3] and EFSA[6]** and has been in use over 25 years. Despite numerous studies confirming it's safety, reports of neurological and behavioural problems have appeared, often after very high doses. Public concern persists especially after induction of tumours in rats[7]. People with phenylketonuria disease should avoid aspartame as it contains phenylalanine which they cannot break down. In the UK,

		Asda is removing aspartame from the "Good for You" range of foods. Children's drinks containing aspartame should be avoided /diluted. Banned in Philippines
iii. **Cyclamate** **(Cyclamic acid)** **(E952)**	Marketed as "Sucaryl" (which is combined with 1 part saccharin to 10 parts cyclamate). Not used in UK until 1995 and found mainly in soft drinks and squashes. Other foods sold containing cyclamates may be imported and include cakes, biscuits, chocolate, jams, cereals, sugar-free	**Cyclamates approved for use by WHO[1] and EFSA[6] but banned in USA since 1970** due to report of bladder cancer in rats fed a blend of cyclamate/saccharin (10 parts:1 part), and of damage to testes in mice fed cyclamate. In contrast, over 75 recent studies failed to show any toxicity to humans and approved for use in over 50 countries. However, safety concerns persist, particularly for 1½-4½

	chewing gum and breath-freshening sweets, as well as pharmaceuticals.	yr children drinking more than 3 beakers (180 ml each) of diluted squashes/soft drinks per day, as the ADI (acceptable daily intake) of cyclamate is then exceeded. The FSA[3] advises increasing dilution of squash/soft drinks for young children to reduce cyclamate intake.
iv. **Saccharin** **(E954)**	Marketed as "Sweet'N Low," "SweetTwin" and "Necta Sweet" (in USA). Used as table top sweetener and found in drinks, sweets, jams,	**Saccharin safety is approved by JECFA[1] and EFSA[6] and in use in over 90 countries but controversial** due to reports of formation of bladder cancer in rats fed high doses of saccharin throughout

	salad dressings, chewing gum, toothpaste, vitamins and medicines.	their lives. Derived from coal tar. Recent research, however, has mainly shown that saccharin is safe for humans due to their different physiology to rats. Generally, evidence "does not link saccharin and human bladder cancer"at the present time. Banned in Canada.
v. **Sucralose** **(E955)**	Marketed as "Splenda". Used widely as table top sweetener and found in soft drinks, ice cream, fruit juices, milk products, puddings, baked goods, sweets, coffee, tea, canned fruit, jam, breakfast snack bars, sauces and	**Sucralose is generally regarded as safe and approved by JECFA[1], FDA[2], and EFSA[6.] It is a recently developed sweetener** (in use in last 10-15 years). In use in over 40 counties including USA and Europe, Brazil, China, Japan, Australia. Safety concluded by FDA[2] from over 110 studies of animals and humans.

	chewing gum.	Even so there appears to be a lack of long-term studies in humans and this coupled with the chlorine content of sucralose has raised safety concerns. The presence of chlorine or chloride in a substance does not indicate toxicity as common salt contains chloride!
vi. **Other sweeteners** **eg.** **"Neotame"** **(E961)** **"Stevia"**	Other sweeteners are being introduced that are artificial, such as Neotame (E961), or natural, such as Stevia (no E number).	Neotame is approved by the FDA[2] and JECFA[1] and has no safety concerns for the EFSA[6]. Neotame is made from aspartame (see above) so similar safety concerns apply. **Stevia** is naturally derived from a plant but even so is not approved in USA or Europe. **NOTE:** because a substance is natural **does not guarantee** its safety.

1. JECFA is World Health Organisation (WHO) Expert Committee on Food Additives.

2. FDA is US Food and Drug Administration (**www.cfsan.fda.gov/~dms/fdsweet.html**)

3. FSA is Food Standards Agency, UK (**www.food.gov.uk**)

4. See reference 37.

5. **http://www.cspinet.org/reports/asekquot.html**

6. EFSA is the European Food Safety Authority (**www.efsa.europa.eu**)

7. See reference 38.

BOTTOM LINE ON ARTIFICIAL SWEETENERS:

- A huge range of foods and drinks contain artificial sweeteners so they are difficult to avoid.

- Many foods containing sweeteners are highly processed and of low nutritional value i.e. junk foods such as soft drinks, cakes and sweets.

- Of concern is the fact that children and teenagers consume particularly high levels of artificially sweetened junk foods and therefore ingest high doses of these additives.

- Food, drink and medicines containing artificial sweeteners are not recommended for babies (and actually banned in baby foods) and very young children (less than 3 yr) as they have rapidly developing bodies which may be particularly vulnerable to any bad effects.

- Many artificial sweeteners are often used in combinations such as **"Sweet'N Low"**, which is a mixture of acesulfame and aspartame, and widely used in coffee shops.

- All ADIs (acceptable daily intakes) are calculated for each additive when used alone but evidence indicates that mixtures of additives, such as sweeteners, may be more toxic (see Chapter 6 of IYL "The Cocktail Effect").

- Most "diet", "light" or "zero" products contain artificial sweeteners. The public is being exposed to a high-powered advertising campaign trying to promote these chemical mixes to gullible children and adults.

5. FLAVOUR ENHANCERS AND FLAVOURINGS

As mentioned above (see page 81), **2600 flavourings** are used in foods and drinks in the European Union but have not been given E numbers since the majority have **not been tested for safety**. Many food labels mention the addition of flavourings but fail to identify them. The European Food Safety Authority (**www.efsa.europa.eu**) intends to rectify this by evaluating the safety of all flavourings. Flavour enhancers intensify and enhance flavours of food without necessarily having a taste of their own. One such flavour enhancer is Monosodium Glutamate (MSG) or 'Hydrolyzed Vegetable Protein,' as it is sometimes labelled on food. MSG is widely used, has received much attention and has also been given an E number, E621.

Monosodium glutamate (E621)

Foods present in: Processed food including sausages, pies, sauces, soups, crisps, stock cubes, noodles, Chinese food, tin foods, fast foods, ready meals and some cheeses.

Safety concerns and possible health effects: MSG has been regarded as safe by JECFA[1], FDA[2] and EFSA[3] when consumed at an approximate average daily intake of up to 10g/day. In addition, no mutagenicity (cancer potential) has been reported. However, many consumers have reported adverse side effects including the "Chinese Restaurant Syndrome" characterized by headache, throbbing of the head, dizziness, nausea, sweating, flushing, wheezing, burning or tingling sensations over parts of the body, as well as chest pain, and back pain. Many of the side effects of MSG are regarded as unproven.

There is, however, some evidence of adverse effects of MSG. For example, it has recently been shown that MSG enhances liver damage induced by trans fatty acids[4] (see Chapter 3 of IYL, Table 1) and may be linked to obesity by enhancing food intake[5]. Also, it has been shown that MSG can induce oxidative stress which could potentially damage organs such as testes as well as DNA, although levels of MSG given to animals were very high. Finally, MSG is chemically similar to glutamate, one of the brains messenger molecules. It may well be able to cross into the developing brains of newborns and young children and possibly cause damage. The Co-op supermarket has banned MSG from its own label foods and many food producers no longer add MSG to their baby foods.

1. JECFA is World Health Organisation (WHO) Expert Committee on Food Additives

2. FDA is US Food and Drug Administration (www.cfsan.fda.gov/~dms/fdsweet.html)

3. EFSA is the European Food Safety Authority (www.efsa.europa.eu)

4. See reference 39.

5. See reference 40.

6. TRANS FATS (HYDROGENATED FATS)

See Chapter 3 of IYL for details of health concerns.

SUMMARY AND HOW TO REDUCE ADDITIVES IN YOUR DIET

- Thousands of foods and drinks contain additives so it is virtually impossible to entirely eliminate all of these from your diet.

- Many of these additives are not essential but purely added to improve colour or taste of food lost during processing.

- Because an additive has been deemed "safe" does not mean that it is good for you. Many **highly processed foods** with lots of colourants, flavourings and swee- teners contain very few ingredients of any value to the body.

- Understand that safe levels of additives (the ADI or acceptable daily intakes) are calculated for each additive when used

on its own but mixtures of additives, found in many products, may interact and **greatly magnify their toxicity/side effects** (see Chapter 6 of IYL, "The Cocktail Effect").

- Reduce or avoid food additives especially if you or your family have young children or have other members suffering from allergies (see: www.hacsg.org.uk for advice) or are pregnant.

- Unborn babies and young children with rapidly developing bodies will be **particularly vulnerable** to any harmful effects of additives.

- Check medicines and vitamins for young children as these may contain additives banned from foods.

- Avoid sulphite (E220-228) and benzoate (E21-214) preservatives as well as artificial colourants (Table 1, above) as this may help reduce allergic responses.

- Dilute squash/soft drinks for young (less than 4.5 yr) children to reduce cyclamate sweetener intake.

- For details of what additives are present in children's foods consult **www.netmums.com/food/Action_on_Additives.992** and **www.foodcomm.org.uk/parentsjury/add_2.htm**

The easiest way of avoiding additives is to drink water, buy locally grown fresh fruit and vegetables, and read food labels to find out what chemical additives are present in your food. A limited number of organic foods are also recommended

(see Chapter 1)

- Organic food is much safer with only 36 additives allowed as opposed to 100s or even 1000s (if you include flavourings) in non-organic food.

- **The good news is that** Sainsbury, Marks and Spencer, Tesco and Asda are removing many additives from their **own brand products**. Britvic is removing sodium benzoate out of drinks aimed at children such as some of the Robinson's range.

- However, these supermarkets **still import foreign foods with dangerous additives**. For example, Sainsbury's own brand pasta is free of trans fats and yet they still sell Italian pasta with trans fats labelled-WHY?

- Beware the terms "healthy" and "natural" found on labels. To check the flavourings in a drink/food look at the label and if it contains real fruit extract then it is natural but if it contains a list of chemicals then it is artificially flavoured.

- Finally, although controversial, products with artificial sweeteners might encourage you to eat more/consume more calories, and put on weight.

The next book in the series is:

It's Your Life – Avoid the Cocktail Effect of Harmful Chemicals in Your Body

For the complete guide to a healthy life:

It's Your Life: End the confusion from inconsistent health advice

Reference sources for conclusions

16b. www.foodsafetymagazine.com

17. www.foodproductiondaily.com/news 20/09/2005

18. www.foodproductiondaily.com/news 08/02/2006

19. Sick Of Pesticides Campaign:
www.wen.org.uk/general_pages/Newsitems/pr_sickofpest
icides23.3.09.doc

20. International Journal Occupational Environmental Health,
Vol. 10, pages 468- 470, 2004.

21. http://www.choice.com.au/articles/a101575p12.htm

22. www.pan-uk.org/index.html

23. www.epa.gov/pesticides/factsheets/ipm.htm

24. www.pan-uk.org/projects/food/index.htm

25. Kroll and colleagues. Reduction of pesticide residues on produce by rinsing. Journal of Agriculture and Food Chemistry, Vol. 48, pages 4666-4670, 2000.

26. www.epa.gov/opp00001 /food/tips.html

27. www.articlebase.com/decontamination-of-pesticide-residues-on-fruit-and-vegetables-317329.html

28. J. Agriculture Food Chemistry, Vol. 50, pages 3412-3418, 2002.

29. www.food.gov.uk/safereating/chemsafe/additives branch/enumberlist

30. Mozaffarian, and colleagues. Trans fatty acids and cardiovascular disease. New England Journal of Medicine, Vol. **354,** pages 1601–1613, 2006**.**

31. McCann and colleagues, The Lancet, Vol. 370, pages 1560 - 1567, 2007.

32. www.moniqa.org/pre/13-Uygun-Food

33. The Food Magazine, March 10th 2007, reported free at news.scotsman.com/gmfood/Alarm-over-banned-food-additives.3353241.jp

34. Ferrand and colleagues, Journal Agriculture Food Chemistry, Vol. 48, pages 3605–3610, 2000.

35. Piper, Free Radical Biology Medicine, Vol. 27 pages 1219–27, 1999.

36. Arranz and colleagues, Toxicology in Vitro, Vol. 21, pages 1311-1317, 2007.

37. Mukherjee and Chakrabarti, Food and Chemical Toxicology, Vol. 35, pages 1177-1179, 1997.

38. Soffritti and colleagues, Environmental Health Perspectives, Vol. 115, pages 293–1297, 2007.

39. Collison and colleagues, Journal Lipid Research, (www.jlr.org/cgi/reprint/M800418-LR200v1.pdf)

40. Hermanussen and Tresguerres, European Journal Clinical Nutrition, Vol.60, pages 25-31, 2006.

www.ingramcontent.com/pod-product-compliance
Lightning Source LLC
Chambersburg PA
CBHW050354280326
41933CB00010BA/1456